A Month of Crystals and Oils:
Enhancing the quality of your life naturally

Raine Mertz

DEDICATION

To my amazing husband Alex for always believing in me and to our wonderful daughter for always inspiring me to be better every day.

CONTENTS

ACKNOWLEDGMENTS

Thank you to all of the highly motivating successful people who have blazed the trail before me, arming me with crucial information to add real value to the world around me. Without their dedication to writing books and teaching classes, I would not have been inspired to devote my life to the wellbeing of others.

A special thank you to Amazon Publishing as well for helping me make my dream a reality by giving me the tools to reach the whole world and help as many as possible.

1 INTRODUCTION

The purpose of this book is to give you a solid foundation to start using crystals and essential oils by implementing four powerful pairings into your daily life. You may be asking, "Why pair crystals and oils in the first place and how the heck do I do it?" Well, the simple answer is that with anything we do in life, the more steps we take to ensure success, the better the outcome.

Look at Robert G. Allen, the bestselling author. The chances of a first time author making it on any bestseller list, (let alone the New York Times Bestseller list), for any length of time is astronomical. But, that's exactly what he did! And, he stayed there for quite a while. He took the extra steps to ensure his success when he wrote his first book *Nothing Down*. It's up to each one of us to take the extra steps necessary to truly succeed in life.

I would like to add that he mentions in his book *Creating Wealth* that he keeps a large piece of Pyrite on his desk. He looks at it when he considers business deals. According to him, it's in reference to fool's gold versus real gold. But, let's just consider the fact that Pyrite is associated with wealth and abundance and Mr. Allen is indeed a millionaire (and a generous one at that). His story is fascinating if you take the time to read it, but I digress...

When you add crystals and essential oils to your daily life, you are adding more layers that can help enrich your life in a deeper and more effective way. This is how you start to ensure your personal success. If one tool is effective, multiple tools will get you there more efficiently and in less time. My hope is that this book will inspire you to incorporate even more crystals, oils, and other healing modalities into your life so that you can truly manifest success in every situation! *Nothing in this book should be taken as medical advice.

On to the how the heck do I do it part...

2 PREPARING ESSENTIAL OILS AND CRYSTALS

Essential Oils

Using essential oils is a fairly straightforward process. First of all, keep them out of the reach of children. As with anything, there can be exceptions and it's entirely up to you whether you want to research and pursue that path, but those uses are not covered in this book.

Always ensure that your oils are properly diluted. When in doubt, go for about ten drops in a 15ml roller bottle filled the rest of the way with your favorite carrier oil.

It's a good idea to store your oils in easily accessible containers such as roller bottles, droppers, spray bottles; whatever is going to make them most convenient for your lifestyle. It's been my experience that if it's not easy to use, it will just sit on the shelf and you can't receive the amazing benefits of oils if they just sit on the shelf. You can easily find a variety of bottles online and in local health stores. Ensure that they are glass and preferably not clear. Excessive exposure to sunlight can damage certain oils, so in my opinion, it's best to be on the safe side by just using amber or cobalt blue bottles for all of your oils.

One last point to keep in mind is to label your bottles! There are few things worse than thinking that you are about to put lavender on your face and ending up with peppermint oil around your nose and eyes. Trust me, it burns. Just learn from my mistake and let's leave it at that, shall we?

Now for Crystals

Crystals actually have a few more steps involved in their use, but the results are well worth it. Crystals work with vibrations. This means that they actually absorb the energy around them from the people that they come in contact with, as well as surrounding areas. Because of this, it is crucial to cleanse them before you start using them. After your initial cleansing, I recommend you cleanse them at least once a month, more if you're using them daily.

When you pick out your crystals, it's ideal if you are able to touch and feel them before you buy them. You will notice that certain ones will resonate with you and others won't, even when they are all the same type of crystal. Unfortunately we live in a time where counterfeits run rampant, so ensure that you are getting your crystals from a reputable supplier or a certified energy healer. Look for someone that can not only assure you that they are authentic, but also understands the importance of handling crystals before choosing one (or more realistically, before the crystal chooses you.)

There are many different ways to cleanse your crystals. We're only going to look at a few of the methods here. Feel free to use the one that resonates most with you as the following are equally effective at thoroughly cleansing your crystals of any residual energy.

1. **Salt water**. This is a simple go-to method that works with any crystal that is not water soluble. (If you don't know if this applies to your crystal, a quick online search will give you a clear answer that will put your concerns to rest.) To use this method, just mix about a teaspoon of sea salt with a cup of water and literally clean your crystal. This will clear all energy away, giving you a clean slate.
2. **Smudging**. For those of you who are not familiar with smudging, it is using a sage

stick by lighting one end of it and allowing the smoke to surround and permeate whatever you are trying to cleanse. This practice has been around for ages, and interestingly enough, science has now confirmed that burning sage actually removes impurities from the air. So, it is effective at both spiritual and literal cleansing. To use this method, light your smudge stick and allow the smoke to surround the crystal for a few minutes. I find it easiest to hold the crystal in the smoke rather than trying to maneuver the sage in such a way as to encompass the crystal. *always use caution when burning anything.

3. **Soil.** This method is very simple and will probably resonate most with the earth signs reading this book. (Obvious right?) You can use a very small area in your yard, a flower pot, or even a bowl filled with dirt. Bury your crystal, covering it completely in soil and let it sit for at least one night.

So, there you have it. Three very different, very simple ways to cleanse your crystals. Now, let's talk about charging them.

Crystals need to recharge their energy to ensure maximum effectiveness. Here are some simple ways to keep your crystals ready to go at all times.

1. **Sun and Moon**. Crystals can be charged by the light of the full moon or sun. Do a little independent research first as some crystals respond better to one over the other. To do this method, the general amount of time is overnight for the moon and at least one full hour for the sun.

2. **Selenite**. A selenite charging plate is an excellent tool for the beginners and experienced alike. Its ease of use makes it a dream come true. Just place your crystals on it to charge them while you sleep. When you wake up, your crystals are ready to go!

3. **Garden**. You can put your crystal amongst living plants in a garden for twenty-four hours to charge them. If you shallowly bury them in the soil, you can use this method to both cleanse and charge your crystals simultaneously.

This final point is crucial to keep in mind when working with crystals. It is imperative to take time with them on a regular basis. As mentioned earlier, crystals can store information. (Look up the piezoelectric effect. It's fascinating and the reason why quartz watches are actually more accurate than your cell phone). The more time that you spend with your crystals, the more your vibrations will complement each other.

This can be as simple as sitting with them in close proximity to you while unwinding at the end of the day. Depending on your goals and current situation, there will be certain crystals that will be beneficial to have with you daily for extended periods of time. For those situations, having your crystal made into a custom piece of jewelry is a wonderful way to display it safely while also getting all of the powerful benefits.

I hope that this has given you a starting point so that you can feel confident as you grow in your experience with crystals. Remember to start small and go at the speed is most comfortable to you. This is an individual practice, not a competition. I know personally how tempting it can be to acquire every crystal you can get your hands on. It is much more effective and less stressful to start with one or two and build slowly.

Now, onto the fun stuff!

3 BLACK TOURMALINE AND CEDARWOOD

This combination repels negativity and negative thinking to allow the good things in life to flow freely. I find it best to start by eliminating the harmful things from your life so that you make even more room for the wonderful things.

Cedarwood is composed of sesquiterpenes which quite literally scrub your cells of bad information, such as negative thinking, addiction, bad habits, and more. This oil assists in healing from traumas and can also encourage quality sleep.

Black Tourmaline is its perfect partner as it physically blocks harmful emissions and radiation and mentally blocks negative thoughts and patterns. Some health benefits associated with it are assisting in detoxification, supporting fat loss, improving circulation, eliminating toxic metals, and supporting the liver and kidneys.

Just keep in mind that you pick up the vibrations that you are exposed to. While this combination is incredibly effective, it is important to guard yourself from negative vibrations and people who would insist on pulling you down. You may find that when you first start working with this duo, some negative experiences or memories may surface. It is normal and will be a lot easier to deal with if you don't fight it. We can't truly find peace and release the things that don't serve us until we acknowledge their existence. It will all be worth it in the end. Let this combination help release you from that may have been holding you back from living the life of your dreams.

A Week

Of Ideas

Sunday

Meditate with your Black Tourmaline by your feet for at least fifteen minutes in a quiet area to start eliminating any negative thoughts or patterns. Visualize a wall of protection around you blocking harmful thoughts and situations. This can be very effective even if you only do it only once, but if you do it on a regular basis, it can give you an undeniable sense of security.

Questions for yourself

1. What were some negative thought patterns that you noticed that you were previously unaware of?

_____

_____

_____

_____

_____

_____

_____

_____

_____

_____

_____

_____

_____

_____

_____

_____

2. How can you shift your focus to turn it into a positive and empowering thought pattern?

_____

_____

_____

_____

_____

_____

_____

_____

_____

_____

_____

_____

_____

_____

_____

_____

_____

_____

_____

Monday

Diffuse Cedarwood at night to allow yourself a deeper and more restful sleep. You can use a traditional essential oil diffuser or simply apply a couple of drops to a cotton ball and place in your pillow case. This can help you process limiting beliefs while you sleep, giving you the opportunity to wake up in a more peaceful and confident state of mind.

Questions for Yourself

1. What dreams or insights came to you while you were sleeping that hold a special meaning for you?

_____

_____

_____

_____

_____

_____

_____

_____

_____

_____

_____

_____

_____

_____

_____

_____

2. What are some limiting thought patterns that you are releasing?

_____

_____

_____

_____

_____

_____

_____

_____

_____

_____

_____

_____

_____

_____

_____

_____

_____

_____

_____

Tuesday

Anoint your Black Tourmaline with Cedarwood and carry it with you to form a mental shield of protection around you. You can carry it in your pocket or purse, whichever is most convenient for you. The important thing is that you keep it in close proximity to you. Take it out any time that you feel you need reassurance and peace of mind. Carrying it with you regularly can also give you access to the wonderful health benefits associated with Black Tourmaline.

Questions for Yourself

1. What reassuring benefits of your Black Tourmaline did you feel today?

2. What are some of the benefits of less harmful energy and radiations that you experienced?

_____

_____

_____

_____

_____

_____

_____

_____

_____

_____

_____

_____

_____

_____

_____

_____

_____

Wednesday

Write any fears, negative mentalities, or overwhelming concerns on a small piece of paper. Apply Cedarwood to the back of your head ensuring that you make contact with your scalp. Meditate for at least ten minutes, actively releasing those harmful emotions. After you finish meditating, burn the piece of paper further symbolizing release. Physically seeing your fears and concerns literally go up in smoke solidifies their elimination in your mind. *Never leave any fire unattended and always use caution when burning anything. It is preferable to burn the paper fireproof container*

Questions for Yourself

1. How did it feel to lift this weight off of you as you released your fears and concerns?

2. What are some other things in your life that you can benefit from releasing?

_____

_____

_____

_____

_____

_____

_____

_____

_____

_____

_____

_____

_____

_____

_____

_____

_____

_____

_____

_____

_____

Thursday

Experiment by placing Black Tourmaline in different areas of your home, such as your bedroom and living room. Make a mental note of which areas feel more effective in eliminating negativity and harmful radiation. Once you have found your ideal space, it may be worthwhile to designate a Black Tourmaline to stay in that area of your home. You may also decide that you would prefer to put multiple pieces throughout your home and even your car. This can be a very effective way to create a sanctuary for yourself and your family.

Questions for Yourself

1. Which areas of your home felt like they benefitted from the Black Tourmaline?

_____

_____

_____

_____

_____

_____

_____

_____

_____

_____

_____

_____

_____

_____

_____

_____

_____

_____

2. How do you think you can benefit from having multiple pieces of Black Tourmaline throughout your home?

_____

_____

_____

_____

_____

_____

_____

_____

_____

_____

_____

_____

_____

_____

_____

_____

_____

Friday and Saturday

Now that you have some experience with this wonderful combination, use your intuition and creativity to find a personalized way to use Cedarwood and Black Tourmaline. Ask yourself these questions. How can I utilize the protective qualities in a personal way that works for me? Where and when do I deal with negative situations and how can I eliminate that stress with Black Tourmaline and Cedarwood? Do I prefer having them with me or near me and how can I incorporate that?

Questions for Yourself

1. What are some exciting uses that you were able to come up with?

_____

_____

_____

_____

_____

_____

_____

_____

_____

_____

_____

_____

_____

_____

_____

_____

_____

_____

4 CLEAR QUARTZ AND THIEVES BLEND

This combination has been scientifically proven to effectively boost your immune system as well as kill bad bacteria! Personally, I use this duo year round to ensure that I am giving my body the extra help that it needs to protect me as much as possible. Doing extra things daily to support your immune system really pays off in so many ways.

I have always found Thieves to be a very interesting blend. The supposed origin of it dates all the way back to the Black Plague. As the story goes, a band of thieves were robbing the bodies of the deceased without getting sick themselves. When they were finally caught, they were offered a reduced sentence in exchange for their secret. Thus the recipe to thieves essential oil blend was revealed. And, it's worth noting that they were using the herbs themselves and essentials oils are more concentrated, so this is a very potent blend.

Clear quartz is an often overlooked crystal. Known as the "Master Healer", this crystal is perfect for giving your body an extra boost to protect it from illness and dis-ease. Clear quartz gives your body the vibrations that it needs to work at a level that is most efficient for true health. It can amplify your energy and thoughts, as well as the properties of whatever it is paired with. It can encourage clarity of thought and purpose in one's heart and mind. This amazing crystal resonates with all of the chakras. It can eliminate energy blockages which can be a major cause of dis-ease.

Use this combination to take your health and wellness goals to the next level! *nothing in this book is intended to be taken as medical advice. You should always consult with your naturopath or physician to see what is best for your current situation.*

A Week

Of Ideas

Sunday

Make a roller bottle of Thieves blend and your favorite carrier oil. Start applying it to the bottoms of your feet and the base of your spine every day to boost your immune system. A good recipe is mixing seven drops of Thieves in a 15ml bottle and then filling it the rest of the way with the carrier oil. Applying this blend first thing in the morning gives your body a boost before you really start to come into contact with things. If you do happen to get sick, start applying it every couple of hours to support your body naturally.

Questions for Yourself

1. What benefits did you notice physically after applying your Thieves blend?

_____

_____

_____

_____

_____

_____

_____

_____

_____

_____

_____

_____

_____

_____

_____

2. What benefits did you notice mentally after applying your Thieves blend?

Monday

Take fifteen minutes in a quiet area to meditate. Either hold your Clear Quartz in your hand or you can lie down with it over your solar plexus. Visualize perfect health radiating from you. As you breathe in, picture breathing in healing white light. As you exhale, see yourself breathing out stale, dirty air. Believe that your body has amazing healing abilities. Allow yourself to be inspired to choose one small healthy activity that you can start implementing daily.

Questions for Yourself

1. How did it feel to picture yourself in perfect health?

---

2. How did you feel after doing the deep breathing visualization?

_____

_____

_____

_____

_____

_____

_____

_____

_____

_____

_____

_____

_____

_____

_____

_____

_____

_____

_____

Tuesday

Diffuse thieves for an hour to remove harmful bacteria in the air of your home. You can either use a traditional essential oil diffuser or apply a few drops to some cotton balls and place in your air vents. You will notice that the air in your home feels cleaner and you may even notice yourself breathing easier. Diffusing Thieves is also an excellent resource for you and your whole family if and when a sickness makes its rounds.

Questions for Yourself

1. What improvements did you notice in the air of your home after diffusing the Thieves?

_____

_____

_____

_____

_____

_____

_____

_____

_____

_____

_____

_____

_____

_____

_____

_____

2. What improvements in your mindset did you notice after breathing in the Thieves while diffusing?

_____

_____

_____

_____

_____

_____

_____

_____

_____

_____

_____

_____

_____

_____

_____

_____

_____

Wednesday

Anoint your Clear Quartz with Thieves and carry it with you. This can give your immune system a huge boost. Having such a powerful crystal in close proximity to you can also help you feel more balanced and optimistic. As your sense of wellbeing is reinforced, you will radiate wellness to those around you, allowing a deeper connection with the world.

Questions for Yourself

1. What benefits did you notice while having your Clear Quartz so close to you?

_____

_____

_____

_____

_____

_____

_____

_____

_____

_____

_____

_____

_____

_____

_____

_____

_____

2. How does your improved sense of wellbeing inspire you to connect with the world around you?

_____

_____

_____

_____

_____

_____

_____

_____

_____

_____

_____

_____

_____

_____

_____

_____

Thursday

Add your Clear Quartz to a relaxing bath with Epsom salts to boost your mental and emotional wellbeing. Set your goal for at least twenty-five minutes. If you choose to use bubbles, make a mental note of where you put your Clear Quartz. There are few things more unsettling than being in a deep state of relaxation in a bubble bath, only to move and feel something unexpected in the water with you that you can't see. Raine's life lesson #1,000,005.

Questions for Yourself

1. What difference in your vibrations could you feel during your bath?

_____

_____

_____

_____

_____

_____

_____

_____

_____

_____

_____

_____

_____

_____

_____

_____

_____

_____

2. What specific feelings of optimism and wellness did you experience during your bath?

_____

_____

_____

_____

_____

_____

_____

_____

_____

_____

_____

_____

_____

_____

_____

_____

_____

_____

Friday and Saturday

Let your intuition guide you and make note of the various ways that you have found to incorporate these amazing tools. Pay attention to which uses make you feel better and more grounded and build on those to allow your wellbeing to really shine. Also experiment with different ways of combining the two. Perhaps making a Thieves spray and adding Clear Quartz chips to the bottle? Ask yourself what ways you think would work best for you and be creative!

Questions for Yourself

1. What are some creative ways that you found to use this healing combination?

_____

_____

_____

_____

_____

_____

_____

_____

_____

_____

_____

_____

_____

_____

_____

_____

_____

_____

5 FIRE AGATE AND YLANG YLANG

This combination is designed to take your passion in your personal and professional life to amazing heights! It's crucial that we take the time to acknowledge and encourage our passions if we are going to truly experience our lives to the fullest!

Ylang Ylang is probably best known as a very popular aphrodisiac, but you may not know that it is also considered an antidepressant. It is effective at keeping you motivated and driven to go after the things you want in life. It can be a wonderful oil to give you extra confidence needed to take the lead in your own life. Ylang Ylang also balances masculine and feminine energies creating a healthy equilibrium, which can assist in releasing feelings of possessiveness and low self-esteem.

Fire Agate is both grounding and inspiring and is known as "the stone of the hero's journey". It brings to light ones true purpose, sparking creativity and strength of will. Use it to find your true passion, and embark on your own unique journey in life. Fire Agate is associated with the sacral chakra inspiring you to have the courage to chase your desires. It reveals the beauty and excitement in life, allowing you to experience real pleasure. This duo is meant to set your inner champion free!

A Week

Of Ideas

Sunday

Meditating with Fire Agate can be a potent way to unlock your inner passion and power! If you're in a relationship, meditate as a couple with your crystal between you to experience the beneficial vibrations of Fire Agate. If you're single, meditate on the powerful vibrations of Fire Agate with a focus on unleashing your authentic self. In either situation, focusing on your Sacral Chakra will amplify your meditation unleashing your true desires.

Questions for Yourself

1. How did the powerful vibrations of Fire Agate resonate with you?

_____

_____

_____

_____

_____

_____

_____

_____

_____

_____

_____

_____

_____

_____

_____

_____

_____

_____

_____

2. How did you fully embrace the feelings of empowerment?

_____

_____

_____

_____

_____

_____

_____

_____

_____

_____

_____

_____

_____

_____

_____

_____

_____

Monday

Add Ylang Ylang to fractionated coconut oil and use it as massage oil for yourself, or you and your partner, focusing on upper body and thighs. Massage is a wonderful way to get to know your own body as well as your partner's body! Adding Ylang Ylang will give you the chance to experience all of your heightened emotions and inner power. (I'm pretty sure this is plenty of information to get you started, and you can use your imagination and take it from here.) *not for internal use.

Questions for Yourself

1. What positive effects did this have on your overall mood?

_____

_____

_____

_____

_____

_____

_____

_____

_____

_____

_____

_____

_____

_____

_____

_____

_____

_____

_____

2. What was your favorite part about the massage?

_____

_____

_____

_____

_____

_____

_____

_____

_____

_____

_____

_____

_____

_____

_____

_____

_____

_____

Tuesday

Anoint your Fire Agate with Ylang Ylang and carry it with you to release the passion for life within you. Having it in close proximity to you can bring out advantageous situations and help you see opportunities that you may miss otherwise. It is advisable to carry this combo any time that you are doing business deals or trying something new. Channel your inner dragon and make life an adventure!

Questions for Yourself

1. What empowering thoughts or feelings did you experience carrying your Fire Agate with you?

_____

_____

_____

_____

_____

_____

_____

_____

_____

_____

_____

_____

_____

_____

_____

_____

2. What were some things that you noticed that you may have previously overlooked?

_____

_____

_____

_____

_____

_____

_____

_____

_____

_____

_____

_____

_____

_____

_____

_____

_____

_____

Wednesday

Write your biggest goal on a Bay leaf and put your Fire Agate on top of it before you go to bed, visualizing yourself succeeding. The Fire Agate will amplify your intentions throughout the night which can help in drawing your success to you. When you wake up, burn the leaf knowing in your heart that your goal is manifesting at this very moment. *Never leave any fire unattended, it is preferable to burn the leaf in a fireproof container*

Questions for Yourself

1. What feelings of excitement are you experiencing while manifesting your goal right now?

---

2. What feelings of accomplishment did you feel burned the bay leaf?

_____

_____

_____

_____

_____

_____

_____

_____

_____

_____

_____

_____

_____

_____

_____

_____

_____

_____

Thursday

Use Ylang Ylang around your chest, neck, and inner wrists to instantly boost your mood first thing in the morning. Using this powerful antidepressant and mood enhancer can make you ready for the exciting adventures ahead. Take your time and really experience the scent and how your body reacts to it. Feel your mood lifting and visualize the wonderful day ahead.

Questions for Yourself

1. In what ways did your mood improve after applying the Ylang Ylang?

----

2. How do you feel that your day was improved by using Ylang Ylang first thing in the morning?

_____

_____

_____

_____

_____

_____

_____

_____

_____

_____

_____

_____

_____

_____

_____

_____

_____

Friday and Saturday

Let you intuition and drive to experience all that life has to offer guide you in creative uses for this power couple. I have only touched on a few uses for them, but this passionate pairing has a lot of uses for ummm...let's just say "adult relationships". As mentioned earlier, just be creative. Look for adventures and embrace new experiences adding to the quality of your amazing life! *external use only

Questions for Yourself

1. What are some exciting uses that you found for this dynamic duo?

_____

_____

_____

_____

_____

_____

_____

_____

_____

_____

_____

_____

_____

_____

_____

_____

_____

6 AMETHYST AND SACRED FRANKINCENSE

This is the combination of awakening and unlocking your higher purpose. Whatever your spiritual beliefs, this combination can be beneficial. Use it to deepen your religious practices and to connect fully with your subconscious and Higher Power.

Sacred Frankincense is one of the only oils that resonates directly with the crown chakra. Grown exclusively in Oman, Sacred Frankincense is known to deepen breathing during meditation, increase intuition, lessen feelings of loneliness, balance emotions, and help heal from grief. Using this oil during meditation and prayer increases your vibrational frequency which can elevate your senses. This makes it possible to be more receptive to the answers that come your way.

Amethyst balances the body's chakras, especially the crown chakra. It assists with emotional issues and encouraging inner strength, wealth, and clarity of the mind. It can help us feel more of a connection when we pray and meditate. There are times when our inner struggles can cause our spirituality to suffer and Amethyst can help us find our inner peace. Incorporating it into your daily practice adds more depth to your spiritual practices which can make them even more enriching.

A Week

Of Ideas

Sunday

Apply Sacred Frankincense to your crown (top of your head) and meditate allowing you to connect to your higher self. Take at least fifteen to twenty minutes to truly open yourself to being receptive of any messages that you receive. Evaluate any thoughts that enter your mind and make note of those that have a special meaning for you. It is often said that praying is talking and meditating is listening. Now is your time to listen.

Questions for Yourself

1. In what ways did you feel connected to your spirituality during this meditation?

_____

_____

_____

_____

_____

_____

_____

_____

_____

_____

_____

_____

_____

_____

_____

_____

_____

2. What specials thoughts or messages did you receive during your meditation?

_____

_____

_____

_____

_____

_____

_____

_____

_____

_____

_____

_____

_____

_____

_____

_____

_____

Monday

Take a relaxing bath with Amethyst and some of your favorite herbs to expand your consciousness and strengthen your connection with yourself. Your conscious and subconscious need to be in harmony to achieve your highest enlightenment. These moments with yourself are crucial for this connection. Think about it like this, it much harder to synchronize with someone that you don't really know. For us to find true inner peace, we need to truly know ourselves. It's ideal to do this self-care ritual on a regular basis.

Questions for Yourself

1. What deeper realizations did you receive during your bath?

_____

_____

_____

_____

_____

_____

_____

_____

_____

_____

_____

_____

_____

_____

_____

_____

_____

_____

2. What specific feelings of inner peace did you experience during this bath?

_____

_____

_____

_____

_____

_____

_____

_____

_____

_____

_____

_____

_____

_____

_____

_____

_____

Tuesday

Apply Sacred Frankincense before you take on any major endeavors. This can allow you to see the larger picture and be able to make the most out of the situation for everyone involved. Focus on win-win and not win-lose. You have a special gift that only you can share with the world and this is an excellent way to open yourself up to the possibilities available to you. Sacred Frankincense can ensure that your conscious and subconscious are at peace in everything that you do.

Questions for Yourself

1. In what ways do you feel a deeper connection between your conscious and subconscious?

_____

_____

_____

_____

_____

_____

_____

_____

_____

_____

_____

_____

_____

_____

_____

_____

_____

2. What were some things that were revealed to you that you weren't expecting?

_____

_____

_____

_____

_____

_____

_____

_____

_____

_____

_____

_____

_____

_____

_____

_____

_____

_____

_____

Wednesday

Anoint your Amethyst with Sacred Frankincense and carry it with you to experience your connection with the entire world. When we realize that we are part of the world and the world is a part of us, we understand that compassion and empathy are the paths to true inner peace. It is quite difficult to harbor ill will towards others when you realize that we are all truly connected. Take time today to love your neighbors and the world as a whole.

Questions for Yourself

1. In what ways do you feel more connected to everything and everyone around you?

_____

_____

_____

_____

_____

_____

_____

_____

_____

_____

_____

_____

_____

_____

_____

_____

2. In what ways are you inspired to show compassion to those around you?

_____

_____

_____

_____

_____

_____

_____

_____

_____

_____

_____

_____

_____

_____

_____

_____

_____

_____

_____

Thursday

Diffuse Sacred Frankincense to further your relationship with your inner self. You can use a traditional essential oil diffuser or you can even add a couple of drops to clothespins and clip them near you. (This works great for car vents too.) Taking the time to directly inhale the aroma of Sacred Frankincense can elevate your vibrations exponentially. Be intentional about it. Don't rush through, but take the time to experience the aroma with your whole body. Follow your positive emotions as they come to you and listen to your heart and mind as they synchronize with each breath.

Questions for Yourself

1. What positive feelings stir inside of you when you breathe in Sacred Frankincense?

_____

_____

_____

_____

_____

_____

_____

_____

_____

_____

_____

_____

_____

_____

_____

_____

_____

_____

2. What enlightening thoughts and insights came to you during this time?

_____
_____
_____
_____
_____
_____
_____
_____
_____
_____
_____
_____
_____
_____
_____
_____

Friday and Saturday

Allow your higher consciousness to guide you in creative uses for this combination. Be ready for new doors to open for you and be willing to receive new opportunities. Meditate for new ideas and inspirations. Think about ways that you can help those around you experience this combination as well. You never know the impact that sharing such a wonderful gift of enlightenment can have. Also be sure to take the time every day to give yourself at least a few minutes of self-love and self-care.

Questions for Yourself

1. What are some enlightening ways that you have found to use this spiritual combination?

_____

_____

_____

_____

_____

_____

_____

_____

_____

_____

_____

_____

_____

_____

_____

_____

7 PARTING THOUGHTS

I hope you have enjoyed your month of crystal and oil pairings. Now that you have established a foundation, continue to research and experiment with different crystals and oils for your daily use. Let your intuition guide you to unique combinations that resonate with you and your personality, as well as your current goals. The possibilities are limitless and you are continuing a tradition that has been used all over the world for centuries.

The model in this book shows you one of the most effective ways of getting to know new crystals and oils as you add them to your daily routine. Trust me, there's nothing worse that acquiring a bunch of new crystals or oils and then not remembering what their attributes are.

Worse yet is having no idea what your new crystals even are because you didn't label them when you bought them. This may not be a big deal if it's only one or two, but when it's multiples, it can be easy to forget at first. Learn from the mistakes of those who came before you and follow the simple steps here. You will be knowledgeable on a multitude of crystals and oils in no time!

Keep getting to know your crystals. You will be surprised at how unique each one is and how they will resonate with you at different stages in your life. The more love and attention that you show them, the brighter and clearer they will shine. This is an excellent indication that you are being a good steward to your crystals. As you continue on this journey, you will learn just how crucial that really is.

If you are looking for a comprehensive guide with information on a wide variety of crystals (far too many to cover here), I recommend *The Crystal Bible* by Judy Hall. This is an excellent resource for everyone and a book that I highly recommend if you're serious about working with crystals.

If you are in need of crystal or energy healing, I would love to help at www.rainesrealm.com and I wish you the absolute best in your future endeavors!

Manifest Success,

Raine Mertz

8 MEET THE AUTHOR

Raine Mertz is the Co-founder and CEO of Mertz Metal and Raine's Realm, whose mission is to help people manifest success through energy healing, education, and one-of-a-kind artisan crystal jewelry. As an experienced Reiki practitioner and Crystal Healer, Raine has devoted her life to the wellbeing of others. She lives with her co-founder and husband Alex Mertz and their child in the U.S. where they are continuously finding new ways to make natural healing accessible to everyone.

To learn more about Mertz Metal and Raine's Realm and see what they can do for you, visit www.rainesrealm.com. Raine routinely offers specialty services for her local and long distance clients as well as the amazing products and one-of-a-kind artisan healing jewelry handcrafted by Alex that can be shipped right to your door.

FOR PUBLIC SPEAKING REQUESTS OR TO SEE IF YOU CAN SCHEDULE A WORKSHOP OR SEMINAR IN YOUR AREA, EMAIL REQUESTS TO RAINESREALMLLC@GMAIL.COM